The Funny Side Collection
The Fart Side
Life is a Gas!
(Expanded Full Blast Edition!)

Dan Reynolds
Joseph Weiss, MD

© 2017 Dan Reynolds •
　　　Joseph Weiss, M.D.
　　　SmartAsk Books
　　　Rancho Santa Fe, California, USA
　　　www.smartaskbooks.com

All rights reserved. No part of this book may be reproduced, reused, republished, or retransmitted in any form, or stored in a database or retrieval system, without written permission of the publisher.

ISBN-13: 978-1-943760-56-5 (Color Print Expanded)
ISBN-13: 978-1-943760-61-9 (e-Book Expanded)
ISBN-13: 978-1-943760-48-0 (Color Print Pocket Rocket)
ISBN-13: 978-1-943760-49-7 (e-Book Pocket Rocket)

The Fart Side: Life is a Gas!

The clear majority of the gasses in intestinal farts, with nitrogen, hydrogen, carbon dioxide, methane, and oxygen contributing 99.9% by volume, are odorless

The minor 0.1% of intestinal gasses that are not odorless includes indoles, skatoles, thiols, sulfhydryls, mercaptans, and aromatic fatty acids.

A surprising percentage of the normal population (predominantly males) profess enjoyment and pleasure with the olfactory stimulation generated by their own farts, but not those of others.

The aroma of a fart can be an indicator of intestinal health.

The gut is the only organ system that can perform its functions without the oversight of the brain.

The Fart Side: Life is a Gas!

Ruminant livestock such as cattle generate more methane from burping than farting.

Indole is used as a constituent fragrance in many perfumes.

The name indole is a portmanteau from the words indigo and oleum.

Indole was first isolated by the dye industry in the treatment of the deep blue indigo dye with oleum.

Indole is widely distributed in the natural environment and can be produced by a variety of bacteria, as a degradation product of the amino acid tryptophan.

Skatole (from the Greek το σχατος = feces), or methylindole, is a mildly toxic organic compound belonging to the indole family.

The Fart Side: Life is a Gas!

Nature harvested jasmine costs over one thousand times as much as synthetic jasmine, which takes advantage of the commercial production of indole.

Skatole is the primary source of the odor of feces, and is produced from the breakdown of the important amino acid tryptophan, the precursor of the neurotransmitter serotonin.

The neurotransmitter serotonin is found in much higher concentrations in the gut, than in the brain.

Tryptophan is an indole derivative and the precursor of the hormone melatonin, the neurotransmitter serotonin, and the plant hormone auxin.

Skatole is an attractant to gravid (pregnant) mosquitos.

The Fart Side: Life is a Gas!

Toilet paper must be ten sheets thick to prevent fecal contamination of the hands with wiping.

Hydrogen sulfide is known for its characteristic odor of smelling like rotten eggs. Surprisingly, women tend to produce more hydrogen sulfide then men.

The small bowel is more than three times as long as the large bowel.

Diet plays a role in hydrogen sulfide production, and cruciferous vegetables such as broccoli, cabbage, cauliflower, and Brussels sprouts are common offenders.

Red meat, beer, garlic, and aromatic spices are other significant contributors to hydrogen sulfide production, which contributes to offensive and odiferous intestinal gas.

The Fart Side: Life is a Gas!

Dried fruits such as apricots are often treated with sulfur products that create odiferous intestinal gasses.

The offensive smell of sulfur products led to several religions ascribing an association between the devil and sulfur.

Activated carbon is used to treat oral poisonings by binding to and preventing the poison from being absorbed by the gastrointestinal tract.

Charcoal biscuits were marketed in the early 19th century as an antidote to flatulence, and are still marketed today for diarrhea, indigestion, flatulence, and as a pet care product.

A hiccup is caused by the involuntary contraction of the diaphragm.

The Fart Side: Life is a Gas!

The scientific study of flatulence and farting is termed flatology.

Flatulence is defined as flatus (Latin blowing) expelled through the anus, as well as the state of being affected with gases in the intestinal tract.

Benjamin Franklin (1706-1790) was a polymath scientist, author, statesman, philosopher, publisher, diplomat, inventor, and humorist. He wrote the following about farting:" Let every fart count as a peal of thunder for liberty. Let every fart remind the nation of how much it has let pass out of its control. So fart, and if you must, fart often. But always fart without apology. Fart for freedom, fart for liberty... and fart proudly!"

Not all taste buds are located on the surface of the tongue.

The Fart Side: Life is a Gas!

Higher methane concentrations in intestinal gas have been associated with decreased gastrointestinal tract motility and constipation.

Tryptophan is one of the twenty-two amino acids, and is also considered an essential amino acid.

Essential amino acids are those amino acids that cannot be synthesized by humans, and therefore must be obtained through the diet.

Because of its importance as an essential amino acid, tryptophan is a common constituent of most protein foods and supplements.

Hemorrhoids are part of normal anatomy, and have an important function in maintaining continence.

The Fart Side: Life is a Gas!

The gut has opiate receptors, which are also found in the brain, and may contribute to addiction disorders.

In addition to being heard and smelled, a fart can be seen if the circumstances are right. In the polar zones, at very high altitude, in frigid weather, or even in a walk-in freezer, dropping a fart from exposed buttocks would look much like the steamy cloud of warm breath on a cold winter day.

Frostbite is a real risk for mountain climbers. For the adventurous climbing Mount Everest, the comforts of base camp at an altitude of 17,590 feet may be the last chance they have for a protected bowel movement. At higher altitudes, there are no shelters so their buttocks are exposed to the extreme winds and weather approaching the summit. Frostbutt?

The Fart Side: Life is a Gas!

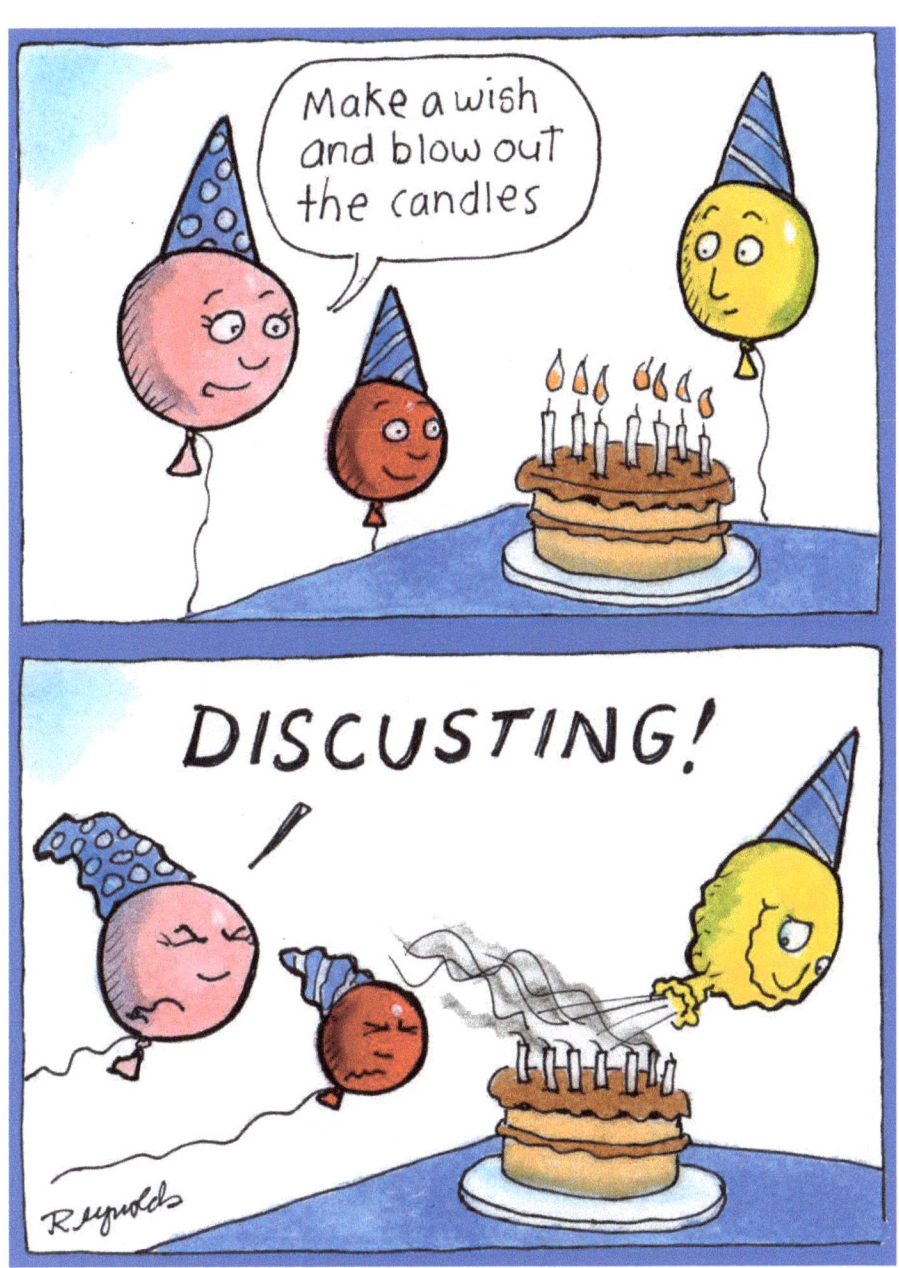

For those wishing to lose weight, the good news with every fart is that you weigh just a little bit less.

Frozen poop stays permanently frozen and does not decompose at high altitude, so there is a growing collection from earlier expeditions to Mount Everest and other summits that is of concern. Climbers are having a more challenging time finding ice that has not been contaminated for melting into drinking water.

The most readily visible of the visual farts occur in the bathtub or when immersed in water.

Over ninety-nine percent of the gas passed in a fart is odorless.

About thirty percent of people enjoy the aroma of their farts.

The Fart Side: Life is a Gas!

As a fart is composed of atoms and molecules it has physical properties, including a mass and weight. Since it is composed of gasses and volatile molecules it is very light, yet the weight is measureable. The total mass of the average fart is 0.0371 grams.

As humans age the production of digestive enzymes decreases so there is a scientific basis for the phrase 'old fart'.

The mechanism of increasing intra-abdominal pressure for a fart is the same as generating increased intra-thoracic pressure for a sneeze. This involves attempted exhalation against a closed epiglottis, and is known as the Valsalva maneuver.

Lactose is the natural milk sugar often found in cheese, ice cream, and processed foods.

The Fart Side: Life is a Gas!

Farts have been recorded with the speed of aroma traveling at a conservative ten miles per hour.

English is the richest language with more words than any other.

The word fart is the correct word to use in the English language, and indeed is one of its oldest words.

The alternative terms for a fart, such as flatus and flatulence, are not originally English words as they have been borrowed from the Latin. In Latin, these words have the general meaning of a wind, or a blowing.

Nitrogen bubbles in a beverage are smaller and longer lasting than carbon dioxide bubbles.

The alphabet of the genetic code of millions of genes has only five letters.

The Fart Side: Life is a Gas!

There is controversy as to the derivation of the word fart. It is thought to have Indo-European roots in the Germanic language word farzen.

The Indo-European word *perd* means fart, and this led to the Latin word *pedere* the verb form of fart, and *peditum* the noun form of fart.

The related Greek word *perdix* referred to a type of bird that made an explosive fart-like sound when it was flushed from the brush when startled. While being incorporated from Greek to Old French it became *perdriz*, then Middle English *partrich*, and finally Modern English *partridge*.

More than twenty-five billion rolls of toilet paper are sold every year in the U.S.

The Fart Side: Life is a Gas!

The word fart is also found in other languages, but there it often has a different and unrelated meaning.

In the Scandinavian languages, the word fart usually denotes speed or motion. In Danish and Norwegian, it is often used in combination with other words that obscures the meaning even more.

For example, in Danish a *fartcertifikate* means a trade certificate.

In Norwegian, a *fart plan* means a schedule.

The Norwegian phrase *stå på fartin* pronounced as stop-a–fartin means ready to leave.

Toilet flush handles have four hundred times as many bacterial contaminants as the toilet seat.

The Fart Side: Life is a Gas!

In then Scandinavian languages the phrase *farts måler*, pronounced as fart smeller, refers to a speedometer.

In Swedish, a speed bump is called a *farthinder*. *Fartlek* is speed training by running at alternate intervals of fast and slow paces.

If you travel on a Scandinavian marine vessel, you may see the control of engine speed labeled as *half-fart* and *full-fart* for half-speed and full-speed respectively. Fart kontrol zones are speed zones.

In Italy, the word *farto* means mattress.

In Hungary, *fartaj* means buttocks.

Ruminant livestock such as cattle generate more methane from burping than farting.

The Fart Side: Life is a Gas!

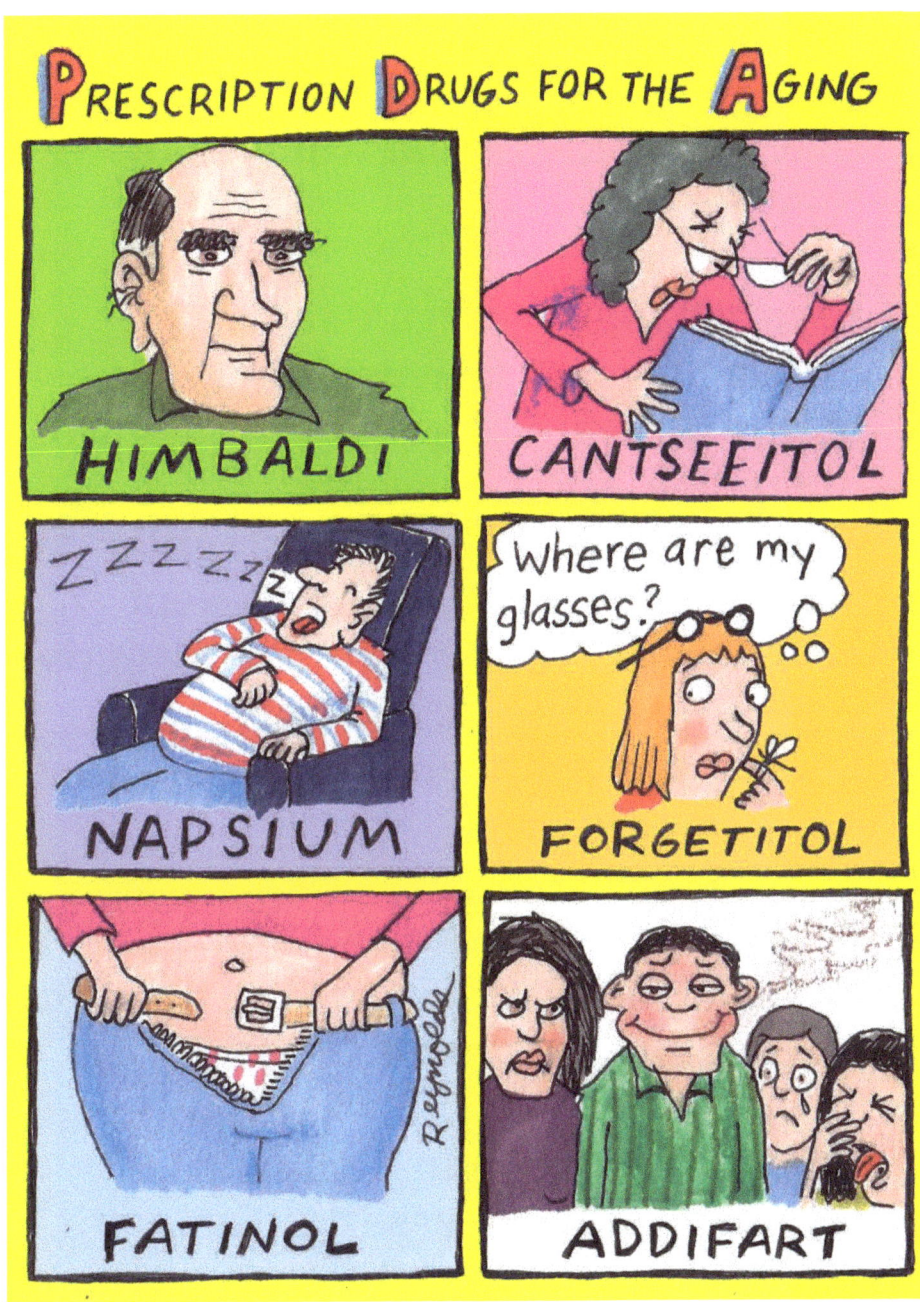

In Poland, if you want to buy a local favorite candy bar with a name that that means lucky, you will be looking for a *Fart* bar.

Several languages have several different words for variations on a theme for which there is only one word in English. The word snow is one example where we have a singular word, but the Inuit, Eskimo, Aleut, Sami and other languages of the native people of the Arctic and northern latitudes may have hundreds of snow variant words.

When it comes to the word fart, the English language is very limited with just the singular word.

American statesman Benjamin Franklin wrote an essay on farts as a practical joke on a scientific society.

The Fart Side: Life is a Gas!

If you smell a natural gas (methane) leak, it is not the methane you smell, but an odorant gas added by the gas company to give notice of danger.

In Germany, a similar word *fahrt* means a journey, trip, tour, or passage. It is often seen in signs that say e*infahrt* (sounds like in-fart) and *ausfahrt* (sounds like out-fart) denoting entrance and exit respectively.

In Spanish and Portuguese fart means an excess of anything, especially food. One of the richest desserts they offer is called a *farte*, which means a fruit tarte in Spain, and usually a sugar almond or cream cake in Portugal.

The gut is the location of over seventy percent of the human immune system, predominantly located in the gut associated lymphoid tissue, or GALT.

The Fart Side: Life is a Gas!

Some of the Russian verbs for the action of farting are particularly colorful. *Perdet'* (to fart with or without sound), *bzdet'* (to fart silently), *pereperdet* (to fart repeatedly), and *nabzdet'sya* (to fart silently to one's complete and utter satisfaction)!

The word fart is one of the oldest words in the English language. One of the most influential dictionaries in the long history of the language is Samuel Johnson's *A Dictionary of the English Language* published in 1755. An important innovation in his dictionary was the use of quotations from literature to illustrate the usage of the word defined.

Air is seventy-eight percent nitrogen, which is poorly absorbed by the gut and when it exits it contributes to burping and farts.

The Fart Side: Life is a Gas!

The name pumpernickel comes from the German language and means Devil's Farts, because the grains in the bread induced potent farts.

While a minority of individuals may have methane present in their farts, methane is odorless.

The individual gasses that make intestinal gas explosive and flammable are hydrogen, methane, and oxygen.

Inflammable and flammable are synonyms and interchangeable words, their antonym nonflammable means the exact opposite.

Most the aroma from a fart comes from hydrogen sulfide, skatole, indole, and aromatic fatty acids.

The most common source of intestinal gas is air swallowing (aerophagia)

The Fart Side: Life is a Gas!

While vegetarians may fart more than carnivores, the aroma is not nearly as pungent or offensive.

Twelve farts per day is a reasonable approximation of the average number of farts humans pass each day, but there is a very wide range of what is considered normal.

The word Fart in northern European languages, including German and the Scandinavian languages, means speed.

The sense of smell requires that odorant molecules from the source material travel to the nasopharynx, and come into direct contact with the olfactory nerve receptors.

The gut is intimately involved in bone health, a role that may involve Vitamin D, calcium, serotonin and other mechanisms.

The Fart Side: Life is a Gas!

Billions of humans are infested and infected with parasites.

Whey is the liquid remaining after milk is curdled and strained.

Absorption of nutrients is conducted by microscopic projections along the lining of the small intestine called villi and microvilli.

A fart contains odorants, as well as transmissible microbes. It is possible to become ill and acquire a pathogen leading to an infection from a fart, much like what can occur with a cough or sneeze.

Pumpernickel (German translation: Devil's Fart) is a heavy dark brown bread traditionally made with coarsely ground rye flour and whole rye berries, which often leads to the intestinal gas giving it its name.

The Fart Side: Life is a Gas!

Like most rye breads, pumpernickel is traditionally made with an acidic sourdough starter, which inhibits the rye amylase enzymes.

Microbes that are associated with mental health and mood disorders are described as psychobiotics.

Without amylase, complex starches such as amylose cannot be metabolized.

Pets de Nonne, also called Pets de Sœur (French translation: nun's farts) are a light airy dessert puff pastry dating from medieval times.

In Western and other cultures, a body may be displayed prior to burial. As the intestinal gas production does not cease with death, and indeed accelerates, gas may continue to escape as an audible fart.

The Fart Side: Life is a Gas!

"I don't usually show this on a first date, but I thought you'd like to see my bear-ass."

Part of the mortician practice is to perform a procedure that seals and secures the anus of the deceased so that the audible release of gas does not occur. Many have been frightened that the corpse is alive when it farts.

One of the most common causes of excess gaseousness is the deficiency of the enzyme lactase, known as lactose intolerance.

Lactase hydrolyses the complex disaccharide dairy sugar lactose, into the readily absorbable simple sugars of glucose and galactose.

Rice is the one starch exception, and rarely contributes to significant gas production.

Enzyme supplements to reduce gas from beans and legumes can be effective.

The Fart Side: Life is a Gas!

With insufficient lactase, the sugar molecule is not metabolized by the digestive system but is instead metabolized by the gut flora, also known as the microbiome.

Lactase deficiency results in gas production and may also give rise to cramps and diarrhea.

Wheat has the other 'distinction' of having the protein glutamate, which contains the nitrogen base product which generates ammonia-like aromatic compounds, that contribute to the aroma of intestinal gas

There are many specific enzymes required in the process of digestion, and deficiency in the quantity or activity of an enzyme can lead to food intolerance.

The Fart Side: Life is a Gas!

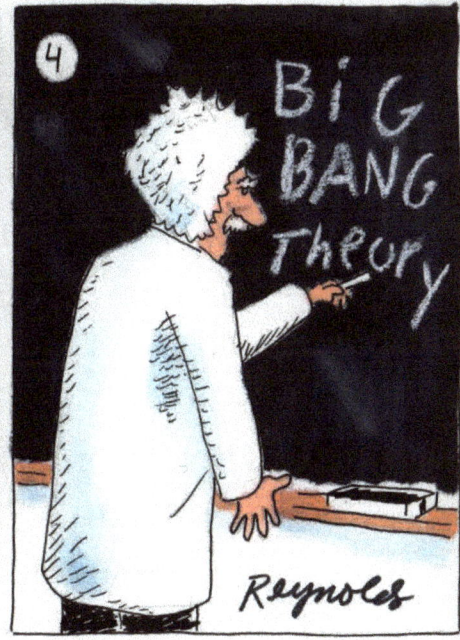

Reflex and heartburn increases the risk of esophagus cancer.

Dozens of hormones, over one thousand and six hundred enzymes, over tens of thousands of species of gut microbes, and over one million genes are just some of the variables effecting the human response to its diet, which also contributes to intestinal gas production.

Air may also be inflated into the colon as the self-practice of the air enema. An air enema is described in the ancient yoga literature as a shake or vat baste.

The advanced yogi may develop anal sphincter control, and control of the abdominal muscles, to create an abdominal suction effect to vacuum air into the lower intestine.

The Fart Side: Life is a Gas!

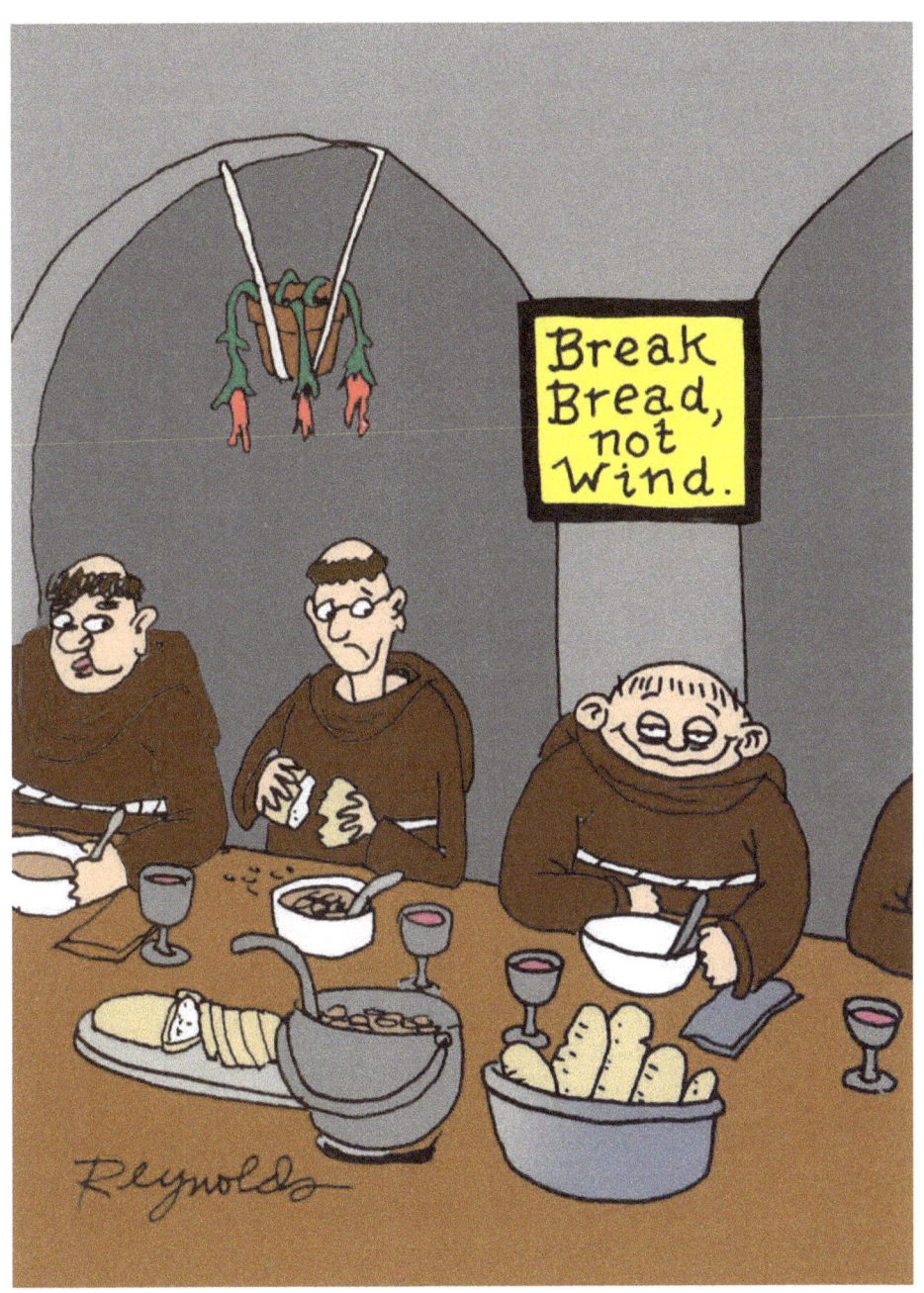

The ability to air fart is the common term for the ability to control the anus and muscles of abdomen and respiration, to cause air to be aspirated into the colon and then released voluntarily as a fart. It is also known colloquially as the ability to butt breathe.

Although usually considered under involuntary control these muscles can be trained, and yogis attain remarkable proficiency.

The air fart and butt breathe technique is known in more enlightened society as an air enema, and has been practiced as a part of yoga colon hygiene for thousands of years.

Gut bacteria produce various metabolites, including the short chain fatty acids butyrate, acetate, and propionate.

The Fart Side: Life is a Gas!

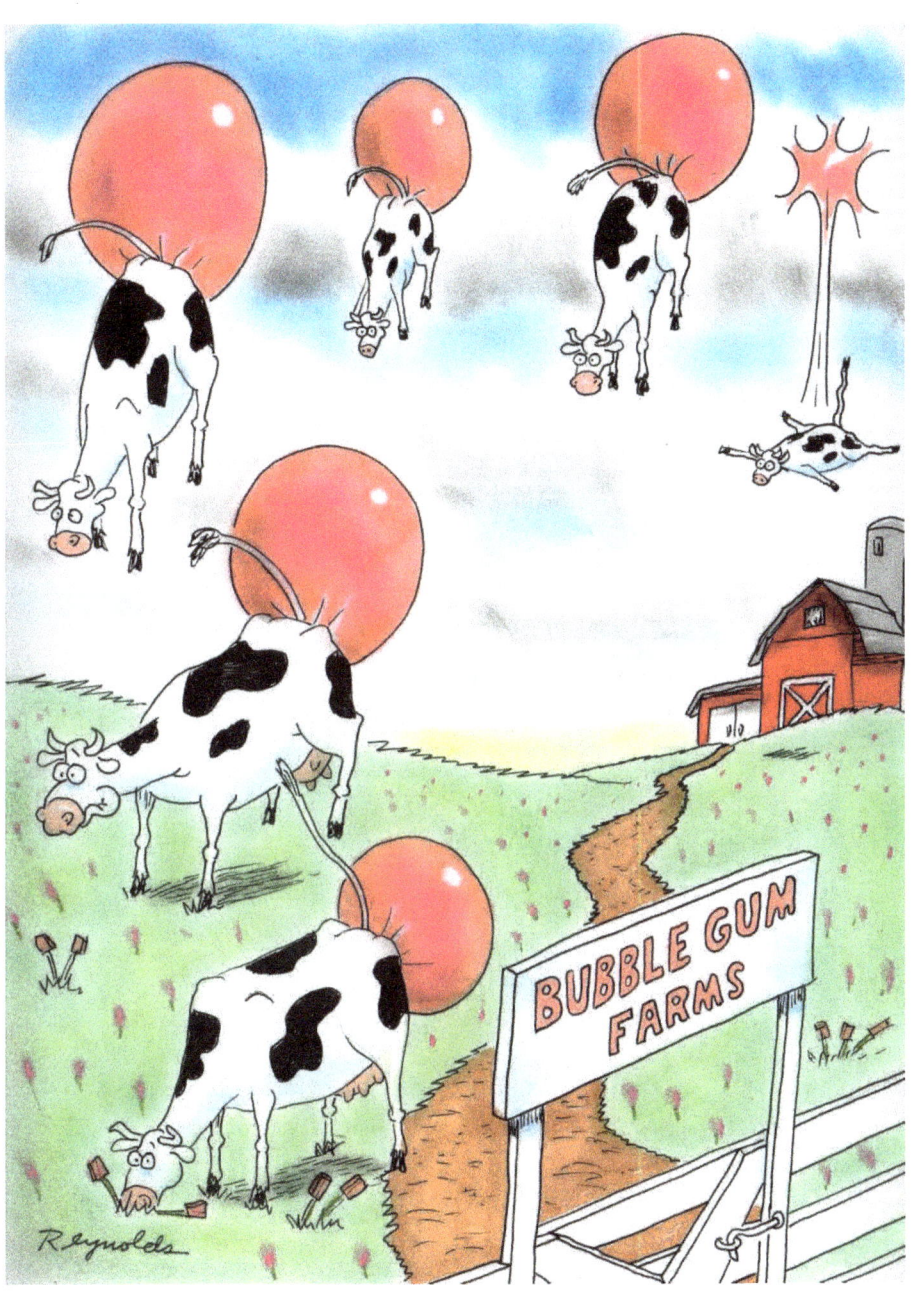

The stomach hydrochloric acid can dissolve metal, and burn skin on contact, but it cannot dissolve plastic.

According to the results of an internet-based survey on farting with over one thousand three hundred participants, over fifteen percent of respondents claimed they could accomplish butt breathing, with the result of being able to fart on command.

At the turn of the twentieth century, the performer Joseph Pujol, under the stage name Le Pétomane, became an international sensation by demonstrating his prowess at butt breathing as a performance art.

It takes several million jasmine blossoms to make one pound of natural jasmine oil, which is two-point-five percent indole, a common odorant found in farts.

The Fart Side: Life is a Gas!

Skatole is attractive to males of various species of bees, who gather the chemical to synthesize hormones that are sex attractant pheromones.

Iatrogenic is the medical term used when a condition is caused by the physician.

Iatrogenic distension with gas is routine in the performance of colonoscopy, endoscopy, and laparoscopy, where tube-like visual instruments are used to examine the internal organs.

In laparoscopy, the gas used to inflate the abdominal cavity, creating a pneumoperitoneum, is carbon dioxide, not air which is mainly non-absorbable nitrogen.

The gut microbiome weighs about three pounds.

The Fart Side: Life is a Gas!

When butt-dialers talk

The carbon dioxide gas is rapidly absorbed by the body and eliminated via exhalation through the lungs. If air were used the large percentage of nitrogen would remain within the peritoneal cavity for an extended period, being slowly absorbed over a period of several days to weeks.

Beano, Bean-Zyme, Say Yes to Beans, and competing products are an enzyme-based dietary supplement that are used to reduce the intestinal production of gas from dietary oligosaccharides such as raffinose, stachyose, and verbascose from legumes. They contain the enzymes alpha-galactosidase and invertase, which are derived from the fungus *Aspergillus Niger*.

The gallbladder is not a vital organ for digestion.

The Fart Side: Life is a Gas!

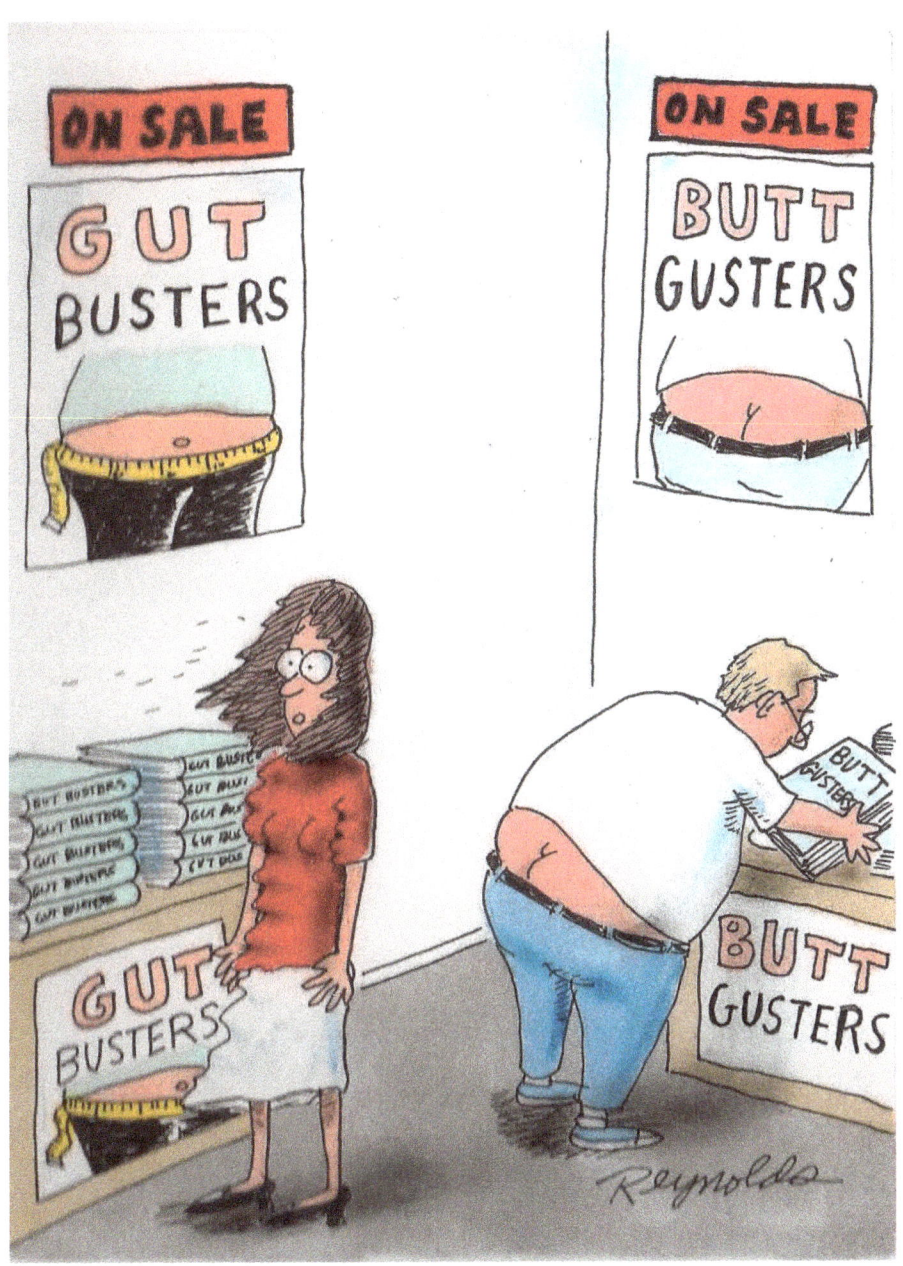

It can take your gut flora up to a year to fully repopulate itself after just one course of antibiotics.

Alpha-galactosidase is effective in reducing intestinal gas, and should be taken with the first bite of food.

Because pets, such as dogs and cats, also release intestinal gas, the enzyme product was marketed for pets under the brand name Curtail.

Because heating inactivates alpha-galactosidase, it is not useful in the cooking process, and must be taken when eating the food.

Higher doses of alpha-galactosidase are needed if large quantities of legumes are consumed, or a substantial period has passed since the dose was last taken.

The Fart Side: Life is a Gas!

Gas production from legumes can be reduced by soaking the beans in water for several hours, and then discarding the soaking fluid. This leaches out some of the complex sugars.

Most people past more than ten farts per day.

Allowing the seeds to germinate allows the bean plant itself to begin to produce alpha-galactosidase. Within twenty-four hours of germination the internally generated enzyme breaks down most of the complex sugars.

Using the herb asafetida can also reduce flatulence, although the herb itself has an aroma that may be worse than the farts that are prevented. The name of the herb appropriately contains the descriptive word fetid.

The Fart Side: Life is a Gas!

The name of the herb asafetida itself gives a clue as to its aroma. Fetida has the same root as the word fetid. These words are derived from the Latin word *foetidus* and *foetēre* meaning 'to stink'.

For every one human cell in the body, there are ten microbial cells.

Beans are being developed that have lower concentrations of complex sugars.

The alpha galactosidase enzyme hydrolyses the complex sugars of the raffinose family including stachyose, verbascose, and galactinol. These are found in foods such as the legumes beans and peanuts, and the cruciferous vegetables cauliflower, broccoli, cabbage, and Brussels sprouts. These complex sugars are the reason the bean is known as 'the musical fruit'.

The Fart Side: Life is a Gas!

Beano, a brand name for the enzyme alphagalactosidase, was marketed by Alan Kligerman of AkPharma, Inc. in 1990. Originally in the dairy farm business, he was the developer of the commercially successful lactase supplement Lactaid. Beano received a US patent in 1995, which has now expired. There are more than fifty competing products on the market. It should be noted that the use of these products enhances the digestibility of certain foods, and increases the nutrients and calories absorbed.

The intellectual concept for a product to reduce intestinal gas was first proposed in the 1780's by the American statesmen, philosopher, humorist, and scientist Benjamin Franklin. He proudly authored an essay entitled 'Fart Proudly'.

The Fart Side: Life is a Gas!

Benjamin Franklin submitted an essay "A Letter to A Royal Academy", suggesting that an award be given to the inventor of a food additive that would make the aroma of flatus attractive instead of offensive. Benjamin Franklin was known as for his sense of humor, and although some thought his proposal was serious, it was written as a satire of scientific meetings.

Simple sugars are produced in the malting process of barley to brew beer. The complex sugars not hydrolyzed or fermented, and thus consumed by the beer drinker, may contribute to its well-recognized ability to increase flatulence. Some home brewers have added Beano to the mash to reduce this occurrence.

The average human eats about 1,200 pounds (500kg) of food per year.

The Fart Side: Life is a Gas!

The use of the prescription drug Acarbose or Miglitol used in the treatment of diabetes mellitus will cause a dramatic increase in flatulence because of its enzyme inhibitor activity.

These drugs are used to treat type 2 diabetes mellitus by inhibiting the glycoside hydrolases, including the alpha-galactosidase family of enzymes necessary for the digestion of many starches.

It specifically inhibits alpha-glucosidase enzymes in the brush border of the small intestines, pancreatic alpha-amylase, maltase, isomaltase, glucoamylase, sucrose, and invertase.

An enzyme is a protein material that speeds up chemical reactions in the bodies of plants and animals.

The Fart Side: Life is a Gas!

Early tests for the cow's moon jump failed due to faulty equipment and methane gas.

Alpha-glucosidase inhibitors are the competitive, reversible inhibitors of pancreatic alpha-amylase and intestinal alpha-glucosidase hydrolase enzyme. Use of these drugs leads to blockage of the digestion of complex carbohydrates in the small intestine, decreasing the amount and delaying the absorption of these sugars.

A diet rich in the amino acid tryptophan can contribute to the fecal aroma of intestinal gas.

Indole occurs naturally in human feces and contributes to the characteristic fecal odor. In low concentrations indole has an attractive aroma, and is also found in the scent of flowers.

Sprouts can provide up to one hundred times more enzymes, vitamins, and essential fatty acids than raw fruits and vegetables.

The Fart Side: Life is a Gas!

At very low concentrations indole has a very pleasant flowery smell and is found in orange blossoms, jasmine, and other flowers and essential oils. It is often used in perfumes.

In the microgravity environment of space, farting results in the body being propelled when the 'digestive gas thruster is fired'.

On the Russian space station Mir, restraining devices were installed on the toilet seat, so the user would not be thrust off the seat with a fart.

Aerophagia is the term for air swallowing, and is a universal and regular occurrence.

Frozen vegetables have higher nutritional value than canned vegetables, but fresh vegetables are best of all.

The Fart Side: Life is a Gas!

Humans swallow on average three to five cubic centimeters, also known as milliliters, (one teaspoonful) of air with every swallow.

Gasses are produced and released in the gastrointestinal tract during the enzymatic digestive processes, as well as with the neutralization of gastric hydrochloric acid by pancreatic and duodenal bicarbonate.

The volume of gasses in the intestinal tract is dependent on the quantity and nature of foods ingested, the body's ability to produce enzymes, air swallowing (aerophagia), microbiome (gut flora), motility of the gut, and transit time.

The transit time, the amount of time it takes for food to move through the system, is partly a function of diet. Adding fiber shortens the transit time.

The Fart Side: Life is a Gas!

A significant volume of gas is swallowed as air, as well as being generated within the bowel. Most the gasses produced are absorbed by the gut, enter the bloodstream through diffusion, and are finally exhaled when the blood flow reaches the capillaries in the alveoli of the lungs. In the alveoli, the gasses diffuse into the air to be exhaled.

Each of the different component gasses have unique properties of diffusion through the bowel wall and into the bloodstream. Carbon dioxide readily diffuses, and enters and exits the bloodstream in solution easily. Nitrogen has a very difficult time diffusing through the gut wall, and explains why air swallowing leads to distension and bloating. Oxygen and hydrogen can be absorbed through the bowel wall.

The Fart Side: Life is a Gas!

Although carbon dioxide is the largest volume of gas generated, and temporarily contributes to bowel distension and postprandial (after meal) discomfort, it is the easiest to eliminate from the bowel. It is only a minor contributor to farting and flatulence.

Twelve farts per day is a reasonable average number of farts passed by humans, but there is a very wide range of what is considered normal.

Commercially available products to trap and contain the dispersion of a fart have been marketed with some success. They rely on the adsorptive properties of activated carbon, also known as activated charcoal, or carbo activatus. Activated charcoal has a very large surface area making it a very effective product.

The Fart Side: Life is a Gas!

Activated charcoal is a form of carbon processed to increase the surface area available for adsorption or chemical reactions.

Activated carbon is used in the purification, decaffeination, metal extraction, water purification, and sewage treatment processes. It is also used in the air filters in masks and respirators, filters in compressed air, and to filter vodka and whiskey to remove impurities that would affect taste.

Activated charcoal has also been used in cases of the ingestion of toxins or poisons. It is taken orally to bind to the toxin to prevent its absorption from the gastrointestinal tract.

Adsorb is the term used when a product is bound to its surface, absorb is the term when it is bound internally.

The Fart Side: Life is a Gas!

The home remedy of eating burnt toast for food poisoning was based on the adsorptive properties of activated charcoal.

Activated charcoal is also effective in adsorbing offensive smelling gasses in a fart. Due to its porosity, a single gram of activated carbon can have a surface area more than 500 meters squared, with 1500 meters squared being possible with further refining.

Its adsorption ability varies amongst gasses and liquids, and it is known to be a poor adsorbent of carbon monoxide, which is toxic and odorless. It is particularly effective in adsorbing most of the volatile odoriferous gasses of a fart.

Drinking a cold carbonated beverage will release more gas than drinking the same beverage at room temperature.

The Fart Side: Life is a Gas!

The key to the success of a wearable activated charcoal product is the degree to which the fart cannot escape without having passed through the activated charcoal. The tighter the seal, the less likely for odiferous gasses to escape.

The sitting pad was least effective, trapping about twenty percent of gasses. Underwear pads ranged from fifty to seventy-five percent effectiveness, while tight fitting underwear entirely lined with activated charcoal were the most effective, but also the most expensive.

Charcoal biscuits were marketed in the early 19th century as an antidote to flatulence, and are still sold today for diarrhea, indigestion, flatulence, and as a pet care product.

The Fart Side: Life is a Gas!

Orally ingested charcoal pills are not as effective in reducing intestinal gas. This may be because the adsorptive capacity of the activated charcoal is fully utilized before it finally gets to the colon, where its gas adsorbing properties are most needed.

Fortunately, bismuth products do provide a significant advantage by binding to the odiferous sulfur compounds, and preventing them from contributing their offensive odor.

The sulfur hydrogen functional group may also be referred to as a thiol group or a sulfhydryl group. Thiols are also referred to as mercaptans.

Antibiotics, designed to eliminate a pathogen, bacteria causing illness, also frequently eliminates the good bacteria of the human microbiome, along with the pathogen.

The Fart Side: Life is a Gas!

The term mercaptan (Latin meaning 'capturing mercury') is used because the thiolate group bonds so strongly with mercury compounds.

The bacteria of your colonic flora generate gas which collect in the bowel. They are joined with the air swallowed throughout the day and night, particularly at meals, and contribute to farting.

The word fart may have originated as an onomatopoeia, a word that phonetically imitates the sound of the event it describes.

It may also have been derived from the word partridge, as the bird makes a similar sound when it is disturbed in its natural habitat and takes flight.

Over four billion people around the world never use toilet paper.

The Fart Side: Life is a Gas!

Pineapple contains the protease enzyme bromelain, which breaks down protein and can be used as a meat tenderizer.

Lighting a cow manure patty is an unsafe way to demonstrate that they are flammable.

Humans who overeat carrots develop skin carrot color pigmentation because of carotenemia, excessive carotenoids in the blood.

Over four billion people around the world never use toilet paper.

Worldwide two million people die each year from diarrhea.

The risk of dying from colon cancer can be greatly reduced by routine screening tests.

The Fart Side: Life is a Gas!

Most the human population harbors parasites.

Certain insects can walk on water, because of the physical property of surface tension.

A rare freshwater turtle in Australia can breathe through its cloaca anus equivalent.

Human blood turns bright red when the iron rich hemoglobin binds to oxygen.

The colon is not a vital organ, and people can live a normal life span without it.

The gut is intimately involved in bone health, a role that may involve Vitamin D, calcium, serotonin, and other mechanisms.

The Fart Side: Life is a Gas!

Vitamin B12 is an important dietary requirement, and its deficiency can lead to a variety of dangerous neurological symptoms and blood disorders.

Swallowing solids requires less neuromuscular coordination and is thus easier than swallowing liquids.

Graham Crackers were developed by a minister as a food that would suppress masturbation.

The average cow releases enough methane to power a one-hundred-watt light bulb for twenty-four hours.

The field of study of the gut brain, also known as the enteric nervous system, is called neurogastroenterology.

Too much hygiene may be bad for optimal immune health and wellness.

The Fart Side: Life is a Gas!

Other products such as tobacco (nicotine), marijuana (cannabinoids), opium/hashish (narcotics), hallucinogenic foods (mushrooms, seafood), can have rapid and dramatic effects on brain function.

Toxins can have dramatic and fatal effects within minutes to days (e.g. Castor beans - ricin, apricot pits - cyanide, puffer fish tetrodotoxin, grain mold - aflatoxin, etc.)

Food can dramatically effect mood. Fat can increase feelings of happiness and pleasure due to the release of dopamine. Carbohydrate consumption stimulates the release of serotonin improving mood.

In many Japanese people strains of their gut bacteria have acquired the genes for polysaccharide digestion from the bacteria found on seaweed.

The Fart Side: Life is a Gas!

Phytic acid is found in seeds, grains, legumes, nuts, and many other foods. It binds to and prevents the absorption of various minerals, and high phytic acid diets have the potential to cause nutritional deficiencies.

Certain gut flora turn phytic acid into inositol, releasing a nutrient involved in mood regulation and insulin sensitivity.

The growth of pathogenic (disease causing) bacteria in your gut is controlled by the presence of populations of good bacteria, which compete with them for nutrition.

Good bacteria also secrete a substance in the intestines that inhibits the growth of harmful pathogenic bacteria.

Gut bacteria produce vitamin K and the B vitamins.

The Fart Side: Life is a Gas!

The balance of beneficial bacteria can be disturbed by eating highly processed foods that may also be pasteurized further reducing the populations of beneficial microbes.

The beneficial microbes in the gut assist in the metabolism, fermentation, digestion, and absorption of carbohydrates such as starches, sugars and fibers. The gut microbiome converts these complex carbohydrates into forms that can be absorbed easily.

The mouth, including the tongue, teeth, palate, pharynx, and salivary glands are all part of the digestive system. Maintaining good oral hygiene is important in maintaining overall health. Besides regularly brushing the teeth and gums, flossing between the teeth, and regular brushing of the tongue add to oral health, and may reduce cardiovascular disease.

The Fart Side: Life is a Gas!

The tongue and cheek muscles participate in the chewing process (mastication), allowing saliva which contains digestive enzymes to mix and chemically react with the food. This is subsequently swallowed as a bolus.

The pH of our stomach is highly acidic (pH 2) due to the presence of very potent hydrochloric acid produced by the gastric glands. This acidic pH is helpful in killing any harmful pathogens that may have entered the body through foods or fluids ingested

The stomach is protected from the acid by the presence of a protective mucus lining. If the protective mucus is deficient or absent, inflammation and injury may result in an ulcer, which can lead to internal bleeding or perforation.

Stomach acidity decreases with age.

The Fart Side: Life is a Gas!

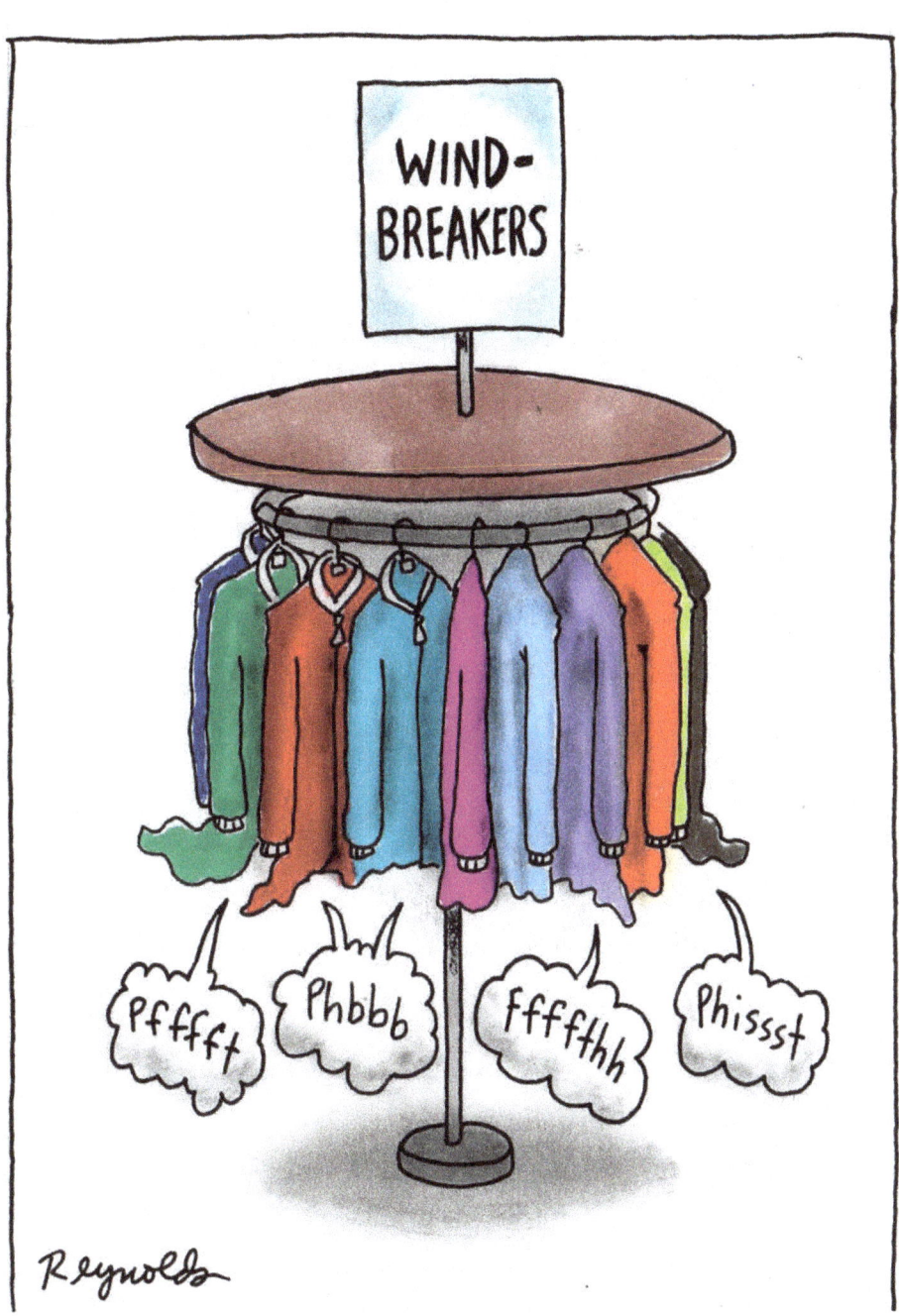

The popular acid suppressing drugs such as proton pump inhibitors and histamine two (H$_2$) blockers have been used to treat peptic ulcers. More recently the cause of peptic ulcers has been identified as bacteria, *Helicobacter pylori*, which is best treated with the addition of antibiotics.

Vitamin B12 is an important dietary requirement, and its deficiency can lead to a variety of dangerous neurological symptoms and blood disorders.

Digestion and absorption of Vitamin B12 requires the presence of intrinsic factor, which is produced in the stomach. Pernicious anemia can occur with the absence of intrinsic factor, and in this condition the vitamin B12 must be administered as an injection, since absorption through the digestive tract cannot take place.

The Fart Side: Life is a Gas!

Gastric acid prevents the overgrowth of the yeast *Candida albicans*, which requires an alkaline environment to grow. *Candida albicans* can be a part of the normal gut microbiome, but can become overgrown in the presence of antibiotics reducing the normal gut flora, eating an excessive alkaline diet, in immunosuppressive disorders or treatment with immune suppression drugs such as steroids, an in the presence of diabetes mellitus.

In the stomach, where gastric acidity reduces the population of bacteria, there may be as few as ten to one hundred organisms in every milliliter. Some microbes, such as Helicobacter pylori can thrive in the acid environment, because they have an enzyme called urease which neutralizes the acid by producing an alkaline material.

The Fart Side: Life is a Gas!

In the small intestine, there may be as many as one thousand organisms per milliliter. Excess numbers of microbes in the small bowel may lead to a condition known as Small Intestine Bacterial Overgrowth (SIBO).

Because our gut microflora changes with age, people over fifty tend to have lower levels of *Bifidobacterium*, an important microbe found predominantly in the large intestine.

We are literally covered in bacteria. For every one human cell in the body, there are ten microbes.

There are three pairs of main salivary glands, and between 800 and 1,000 minor salivary glands. The main salivary glands are exocrine glands which secrete saliva via ducts that drain into the mouth.

The Fart Side: Life is a Gas!

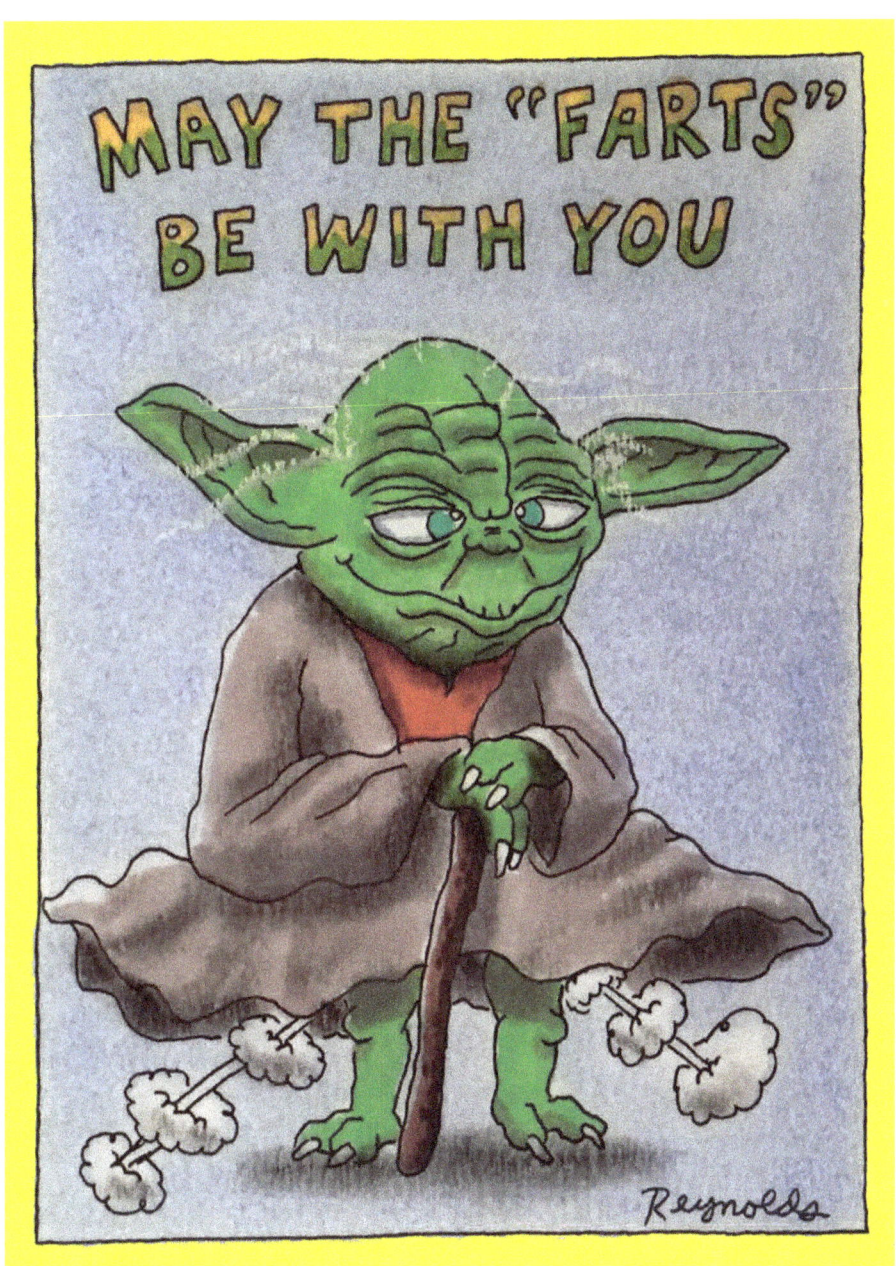

The liver uses cholesterol to generate bile acids, which is one way the body eliminates excess cholesterol.

Bile acids are the detergents found in bile, made by the liver and stored in the gallbladder. The detergents allow fat to mix well with water, allowing the fats to be digested and absorbed. And, just like dish detergent, they make fat mix well with water, and only then can digestive enzymes break down the fat for absorption into the bloodstream.

The body also uses cholesterol to make the sex hormones, like estrogen and testosterone.

Your gut flora actively synthesizes various nutrients: vitamin K, pantothenic acid, folic acid, vitamin B1, B2, B3, B6, and B12, as well as various amino acids and proteins.

The Fart Side: Life is a Gas!

The gallbladder stores the bile secreted by the liver, and releases it into the duodenum of the small intestine when food rich in cholesterol or other lipids is ingested.

The bile secreted by the gall bladder emulsifies fat molecules so that fat digestive enzymes, like lipase, can carry out their breakdown and digestion effectively.

The gallbladder concentrates the bile acid content of the bile tenfold.

Removing the gallbladder does not interfere significantly with fat metabolism as the bile is directly secreted to the intestine.

Some gallstones, made from calcium and extra fatty cholesterols, can be dissolved with bile acid supplements.

The Fart Side: Life is a Gas!

The Funny Side Collection

Dan Reynolds
Joseph Weiss, MD

Dan Reynolds
Joseph Weiss, MD

Dan Reynolds
Joseph Weiss, MD

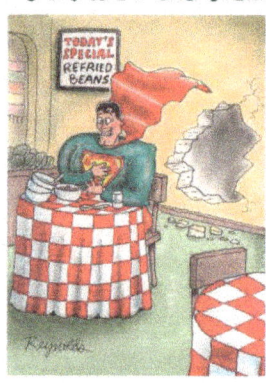

Dan Reynolds
Joseph Weiss, MD

Available in 5"x7" (96 pages) Pocket Rocket! & 6"x9" (122 pages) Expanded Full Blast! print/e-book edition

www.thefunnysidecollection.com

The Fart Side: Life is a Gas!

Dan Reynolds

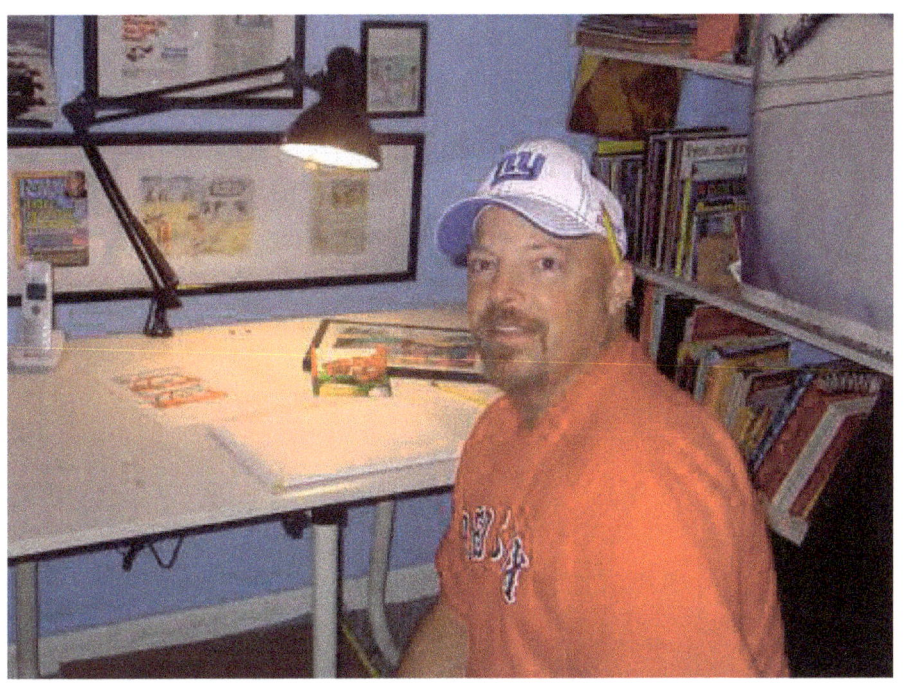

Dan Reynolds began drawing cartoons in December of 1989. He draws and eats left-handed. He plays ping pong and pool left-handed. He throws, kicks and bats right-handed. Like a box of chocolates, you never know what you're going to get, but you will like most of them and they'll keep you coming back. Unlike chocolates, REYNOLDS UNWRAPPED cartoons are not fattening.

The Funny Side Collection

Dan's cartoons are seen by millions of readers across the U.S., Canada, and points beyond all the way down under in Australia. His work is seen in every issue of Reader's Digest (where he is known for his cow, pig, and chicken cartoons).

His cartoons have appeared on HBO's The Sopranos, the cover of a National Lampoon cartoon book collection, and on greeting cards all throughout the United States. His work also appears in many other places as well.

Sign-up for Dan's daily REYNOLDS UNWRAPPED e-mail cartoon for only $12 for a whole year. E-mail Dan at reynoldsunwrapped@gmail.com for details. Dan's website is:
www.reynoldsunwrapped.weebly.com

The Fart Side series and other items are available at:
www.thefunnysidecollection.com

The Fart Side: Life is a Gas!

Joseph Weiss, M.D.

GI Joe is Clinical Professor of Medicine in the Division of Gastroenterology at the University of California, San Diego. He is a Fellow of the American College of Physicians, Fellow of the American Gastroenterological Association, and a Senior Fellow of the American College of Gastroenterology.

Dr. Weiss is the author of several dozen books on health available at:
www.smartaskbooks.com

He is an accomplished professional speaker and humorist, having given over three thousand invited presentations internationally at universities, international conventions, conferences, corporations, resorts, and special events.

The Fart Side series and other items are available at:
www.thefunnysidecollection.com

"Dr. Joseph Weiss' books provide an informative and entertaining approach to sharing insights about our digestive system and wellbeing." **Deepak Chopra, MD**

"Joseph Weiss, M.D. has a gift for books that are uniquely informative and entertaining. **Jack Canfield** Coauthor of the Chicken Soup for the Soul® series

The Fart Side: Life is a Gas!

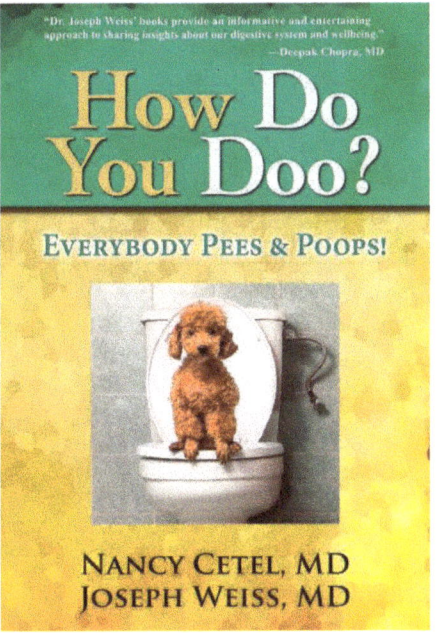

www.smartaskbooks.com

The Funny Side Collection

www.smartaskbooks.com